Testosterone: The Hormone for Strong Bones, Sex Drive and Healthy Menopause

Dr. Susan's Healthy Living
drsusanshealthyliving.com

I0427988

Facebook.com/DrSusanRichards
drsusanshealthyliving@gmail.com
(650) 561-9978

Mention of specific companies or products in this book does not suggest endorsement by the author or publisher. Internet addresses and telephone numbers for resources provided in this book were accurate at the time it went to press.

ISBN 978-1512225969

Note

The information in this book is meant to complement the advice and guidance of your physician, not replace it. It is very important that any person who has medical problems be evaluated by a physician. If you are under the care of a physician, you should discuss any major changes in your regimen with him or her. Because this is a book and not a medical consultation, keep in mind that the information presented here may not apply in your particular case. In view of individual medical requirements, new research, and government regulations, it is the responsibility of the reader to validate health practices and treatments with a physician or health service.

Table of Contents

1

The Benefits of Testosterone for the Female Body

Most women want to enjoy their lives with strength, vitality, and vigor. We want to maintain a zest for life and be able to participate in our favorite activities, including sex. We also want to be able to think clearly and remember facts and events. No one relishes the idea of becoming infirm or losing the faculties needed to fully participate in our favorite activities. We want to maintain a vital and active life as we become older.

This becomes more difficult to achieve once we pass through menopause and the levels of our sex hormones begin to greatly diminish. Most of us are concerned about our bodies' need for estrogen and progesterone and there is much focus on finding good replacement therapy for these essential hormones. Yet, our third sex hormones, testosterone, is equally important in supporting the quality of our lives.

I have always felt that testosterone is often misunderstood, and even ignored, by women. While most often associated with men, muscles, and aggression, testosterone is a critical hormone for women as well. Like estrogen and progesterone, testosterone is critical for your reproductive health. It plays a key role in several other health functions, including heart health and the strength of your tissues, and your mood. It plays a key role in drive and assertiveness. It also supports your energy, mental agility, mood, outlook on life, and sex drive.

If you are like most women, you probably don't spend much time thinking about your testosterone levels. While testosterone is typically thought of as a "male hormone, it is just as critical to your health as the more feminine hormones estrogen and progesterone. You simply produce testosterone in much smaller amounts.

In this book, I am going to take a closer look at this "male" hormone and discuss its importance for the female body and how it benefits women's health. I will provide you with important information on how to evaluate your own testosterone levels as well as the medical testing for this important hormone. Most importantly, I will be sharing with you many powerful natural therapies to not only support your own level of testosterone but also to combat symptoms that are found with testosterone deficiency. These incredible therapies will help to restore your zest for life, energy, and sense of well-being as well as reduce symptoms of menopause and stren-gthen your body.

In the following chart, I list a summary of the benefits of testosterone for our body, mind and emotions. I will be discussing these benefits in more detail in the following chapters.

Benefits of Testosterone

Peak-Performance Benefits for Women
- Increased physical vitality and stamina (restores energy)
- Strengthened determination and perseverance in pursuing goals (includes enhanced assertiveness and libido)
- Increased ability to get along with other people (balances mood)

Health Benefits for Women
- Relieves menopausal symptoms such as hot flashes, nervousness, and vaginal dryness
- Relieves anxiety and depression
- Helps prevent osteoporosis
- Helps relieve arthritis

2

How Sex Hormones Benefit Peak Performance and Health

In this chapter, I discuss the topic of sex hormones in general. All of our major sex hormones, testosterone, estrogen, and progesterone, share certain characteristics in terms of how they function in the body and how they are manufactured by our endocrine glands. If you want to skip this chapter, you can go on to the next chapter to learn important information about testosterone

How Hormones Function in the Body

Hormones are powerful substances that function as the chemical messengers of the body. They are primarily secreted by our glands and released into the bloodstream, where they circulate either to a target gland or to various tissues of the body. Hormones either stimulate a target gland to release its own hormone or directly trigger chemical reactions in the tissues.

The glands of the body (also referred to as the endocrine system) secrete dozens of hormones, which have a multitude of physiological effects on target tissues. Working in concert, hormones initiate and coordinate cellular events, as well as balancing and pacing various physiological processes.

As an integral part of many bodily functions, hormones enhance cognitive abilities, help stabilize mood, and are essential for health, promoting growth, healing, and repair. They play a crucial role in preventing the onset of many ailments, such as cardiovascular disease, Alzheimer's disease, and osteoporosis.

Considering all the functions that hormones influence, it is no wonder that achieving excellence in any area of life is not possible without an optimally functioning endocrine system.

What Are Sex Hormones?

Sex hormones belong to a classification called steroid hormones, which are all derived from cholesterol, a waxy, white, fatty material found in all cells of the body.

The sex hormones are made in the adrenal glands in both men and women. Women also produce sex hormones in the ovaries (a pair of almond-sized glands nestled deep in a woman's pelvis), while men produce these hormones in the testes (two small oval glands located in the scrotum that are also responsible for producing sperm).

Within these tissues, cholesterol is converted to hormones through a number of intermediary steps, leading to the final production of three major sex hormones — estrogen and progesterone in women and testosterone in men.

Both men and women produce the same three major sex hormones but in different proportions. In women, estrogen and progesterone predominate, supporting normal functioning of the reproductive tract and menstrual cycle. The ovaries and adrenals also make small amounts of male hormones, or androgens including testosterone.

Although it is only secreted in tiny amounts, testosterone plays a vital role in the female libido, or sex drive, as well as helping to maintain bone mass. In men, the reverse is true: The predominant hormone is testosterone, which controls sperm production as well as libido. However, men also produce tiny amounts of estrogen and progesterone.

The sex hormones help to determine the physical characteristics of both men and women, such as skin texture, muscle tone, and body shape as well as our emotional make-up.

How Sex Hormones Are Produced Within the Body

Sex hormones are produced through a series of chemical reactions, beginning with cholesterol. Of the total cholesterol in the body, about 75 percent is produced in the liver. The remaining 25 percent is supplied in the diet by foods such as meat and dairy products.

On average, a person's body contains about one-third of a pound of cholesterol (150g), mostly as a component of cell membranes. There is also about 7g of cholesterol that circulates in the blood.

Both the overproduction and the underproduction of cholesterol can lead to hormone imbalances. People who go on stringent low-fat diets may lower their levels of cholesterol to such a degree that they don't have enough to make sufficient amounts of hormones.

For example, teenage girls who go on crash diets often have irregular menstrual cycles, as their body's production of estrogen and progesterone, which regulate the cycle, diminishes.

At the other extreme, people who are obese and eat the high-fat foods of the standard American diet have the opposite risk: Their bodies make too much cholesterol, making them prone to diseases and disorders for which elevated levels of estrogen are a risk factor, including premenstrual syndrome (PMS), fibroid tumors, fibrocystic disease of the breast, heavy menstrual bleeding, and uterine cancer.

Cholesterol is first converted into pregnenolone, a steroid hormone that is the precursor to all the other sex hormones. Because of its precursor role, pregnenolone is considered the "mother sex hormone", thus inspiring its name.

Pregnenolone is then converted into a variety of other hormones, following two pathways. By one route, pregnenolone leads to another precursor hormone, DHEA (dehydroepiandrosterone), which is then converted into testosterone and subsequently estrogen. This pathway is operative in women during the first half of the menstrual cycle, when estrogen is the dominant hormone.

In the second pathway, pregnenolone is converted into progesterone. The progesterone is then converted into testosterone and, finally, into estrogen. In females, this second pathway predominates during the second half of the menstrual cycle, when progesterone and estrogen are dominant.

How Hormones Deliver Their Messages

Each hormone is coded to bind only to certain tissues. The cells in these hormone-sensitive tissues contain specific receptors. When a hormone reaches its target tissue, it binds to these receptors like a key fitting into a lock. When binding occurs, the hormone then transmits its chemical message to the target tissue, causing a change in the tissue.

For example, estrogen is a growth stimulating hormone that causes tissues to grow and thicken, while progesterone is a growth-limiting hormone. Some hormones can cause rapid changes in a target tissue, occurring literally within seconds, while other reactions may take several days, but may then have a continuing influence for days or even years.

Summary

Hormones, primarily secreted by the glands, or endocrine system, are the chemical messengers of the body. They perform myriad functions and are divided into several categories. The series of chemical reactions that produce the sex hormones begins with cholesterol.

The three major sex hormones are testosterone, a primarily male hormone, and estrogen and progesterone, which are primarily female. The two precursor hormones, from which these and all other sex hormones are made, are pregnenolone and DHEA. An adequate supply of sex hormones and their precursors is necessary for peak performance and optimal health.

3

The Production of Testosterone in Women

Testosterone, and all other androgens or male hormones, are sex steroid compounds and share the characteristics described in the previous chapter. They also have a similar structure. They can all be synthesized in both men and women from the waxy, fatty substance cholesterol or made directly from acetyl Coenzyme A, a chemical produced in the liver and made from fatty acids and amino acids.

In men, testosterone is essential for normal sexual behavior; it also promotes the development of secondary sexual characteristics such as facial hair and the lower pitch of the male voice. But beyond its impact on sexuality and appearance, testosterone influences many metabolic activities that affect such fundamental performance factors as energy level and cognitive thinking.

The use of testosterone as a male tonic has a long history. Traditional healers have used the sexual organs and glands of male animals to restore potency in men. These medicines probably contained small quantities of animal testosterone. The search for a male elixir continued into modern times.

In France, in the late nineteenth century, physiologist Charles-Édouard Brown-Séquard injected himself with fluid extracted from animal testicles and pronounced the substance rejuvenating. The use of such substances to treat male impotence became a fad in the first decades of this century; however, it is questionable whether these contained active ingredients or only had a placebo effect. Then in 1934, scientists synthesized testosterone from cholesterol, preparing the way for the development of present-day testosterone replacement therapy.

Women also produce testosterone, at much lower levels than men, in the ovaries and adrenal glands. Like men, testosterone also provides us with a number of important peak performance and health benefits.

How Testosterone is Produced Within the Female Body

Similar to the other female hormones, estrogen and progesterone, testosterone production is also stimulated in the brain, specifically by the hypo-thalamus. The hypothalamus is the master endocrine gland contained within your brain that regulates your production of all sex hormones.

Hypothalamus also regulates other characteristics like your emotions and thirst. This important gland produces a precursor hormone called gonadotropin releasing hormone (GnRH). When it is released, it travels to your anterior pituitary gland, where it stimulates the secretion of the follicle stimulating (FSH) and luteinizing hormones (LH). These hormones then travel to the adrenals and ovaries, where they stimulate the production of the more masculinizing hormones, testosterone and andro-stenedione, as well as the more feminizing hormones, estrogen and progesterone.

Like estrogen and progesterone, the level of andro-stenedione varies throughout your menstrual cycle. The level rises at mid-cycle, when androstenedione is secreted from the ovarian follicle (the structure in your ovary containing a female reproductive cell), and during the second half of the menstrual cycle, when it is produced by the corpus luteum. The corpus luteum is the structure that develops within the ruptured ovarian follicle after ovulation or the release of the egg from the ovary.

Because LH controls the production of the androgens such as androstenedione and testosterone, low levels of LH often correlate to low levels of these androgens. In fact, research has shown that if you can increase your body's production of LH, you can better support your own production of testosterone.

The Availability of Testosterone in Women

A woman normally produces about 0.3 mg of testosterone per day. Total production is about one-tenth the amount produced by men. Production peaks around age twenty, and by the time a woman reaches age forty, it will have declined by about half. After menopause, testosterone production in women is minimal. Most circulating testosterone is bound to sex hormone–binding globulin (SHBG), with only a small percentage that is biologically active. Because estrogen increases the concentration of SHBG, natural fluctuations in estrogen levels, as well as estrogen replacement therapy, can further diminish available testosterone.

Testosterone's Role in Your Body

Testosterone plays an important role in normal female sexual development. The initiation of menstruation and puberty is, in part, triggered by testosterone production. Additionally, testosterone stimulates libido. Levels of the hormone rise and decline during the menstrual cycle to insure that sexual desire increases just before ovulation, when a woman is fertile and chances are greatest for conception.

As with men, testosterone stimulates libido in women. Levels of the hormone rise and decline during the menstrual cycle to insure that sexual desire increases just before ovulation, when a woman is fertile and chances are greatest for conception.

Testosterone also restores vitality and energy levels, helps reduce depression, balances mood and, in part, engenders attributes such as optimism, assertiveness, and aggressiveness that are usually associated with male behavior. Testosterone also benefits female health by helping to relieve menopausal symptoms such as hot flashes, nervousness, vaginal dryness, and the strength of vaginal tissues. It can also help to prevent osteoporosis.

4

How Testosterone Deficiency Occurs

You normally produce about 0.3 mg of testosterone per day. Total production is about one-tenth the amount produced by men. Production peaks around age 20, and by the time you reach age 40, it will have declined by about half. Additionally, older women exhibit a circadian variation in their androstenedione (and thus testosterone) levels, with the greatest concentration mid-morning and the least mid- to late-afternoon. This is due to adrenal activity, which affects (in part) testosterone production.

As is the case with all sex hormones, testosterone production from both the adrenal glands and the ovaries also decreases after menopause. Most circulating testosterone is bound to sex hormone-binding globulin (SHBG), with only a small percentage that is biologically active. Because estrogen increases the concentration of SHBG, natural fluctuations in estrogen levels, as well as estrogen replacement therapy can further diminish available testosterone.

Interestingly, postmenopausal women seem to express the physical signs of their testosterone production more after menopause than before. For example, subtle signs of masculinization many occur after post-menopause, which can be distressing for many women. This can include hair growth on the chin and chest, thinning hair on the scalp, and more sparse pubic hair. The reason for this is that while testosterone production drops after menopause, estrogen levels drop even more drastically. Normally, your high levels of estrogen block this male pattern of hair growth (or loss) from occurring. However, after menopause, this unusual growth (or loss) of hair is stimulated by the action of the male hormones on the follicle

How Diet, Lifestyle, and Health Affect Testosterone Levels

As we have just discussed, the aging process affects testosterone levels in both men and women, but testosterone levels are also sensitive to various environmental factors such as diet, alcohol use, lifestyle habits such as smoking, stress levels, and a person's general state of health. Poor lifestyle habits can negatively impact testosterone production as well as sperm count.

Eating a typical American high-fat diet can alter testosterone levels. This correlation was demonstrated in a study published in *Modern Medicine*.

Eight healthy men, ages twenty-three to thirty-five, were given a daily milk shake containing 800 calories, 57 percent of which was fat. The researchers found that following the high-fat meal, blood levels of testosterone dropped by about 30 percent. How much caffeine and alcohol a person consumes will also affect testosterone levels. The effect of caffeine on testosterone levels in women was investigated in a large study published in 1996 in the *American Journal of Epidemiology*. Women who had more than two cups of coffee or four cans of caffeinated soda per day experienced a decline in testosterone levels.

Stress

Stress is also associated with diminished hormone levels, as evidenced in a study appearing in the *Journal of Internal Medicine*. The study examined 439 men, all aged 51, and found that chronic psychosocial stresses such as tense, difficult working conditions, painful thoughts, and sad feelings were associated with a low testosterone level. The researchers suggested that chronic stress contributed to premature aging.

Physiological Factors

Having a low level of HDL cholesterol, which performs the function of transporting hormones, can impair the body's ability to produce testosterone. Poor digestive function can also be a limiting factor.

The ability of the body to absorb certain substances such as fat molecules and fragments of protein from which hormones are manufactured affects the quantity of testosterone that the body can produce. How well the liver is able to break down toxins and metabolize hormones will also impact testosterone levels.

Symptoms of Testosterone Deficiency

Even the small amount of testosterone that a woman produces can have a significant effect on her performance and influence her quality of life. If levels are below normal, you can experience a wide range of emotional symptoms, including decreased energy, depression, and anxiety. You will also notice a few physical effects as well, such as osteoporosis, loss of libido, and insomnia. I will be discussing the symptoms of testosterone deficiency in the next three chapters.

5

Testosterone and Peak Performance in Women

Even the small amount of testosterone that a woman produces can have an effect on her performance and influence her quality of life. It's not just men who receive a pick-me-up and enhanced strength from testosterone. Women benefit too! As in men, testosterone increases our energy, enhances mood and imparts a sense of well-being, and stimulates assertiveness and libido in women. These are all great quality of life benefits. These effects have been observed in women who have taken testosterone replacement to restore natural levels of the hormone. I want to share some of this amazing research with you.

Physical Vitality and Stamina

Various studies have demonstrated that women taking a hormone replacement that includes estrogen *and* testosterone experience a greater level of energy than women on estrogen alone.

In a study published in *The American Journal of Obstetrics and Gynecology*, forty-three women had received a total hysterectomy, including removal of their ovaries. As the ovaries make one-third of the testosterone in the female body, their removal causes a significant decline in testosterone production.

The women were divided into four groups and given combined estrogen and testosterone, one or the other of the hormones alone, or a placebo. A treatment was administered for three months, followed by a differing treatment for another three months. There was also a control group of ten women who underwent hysterectomy but retained their ovaries.

The women receiving testosterone therapy, alone or with estrogen, and the women with ovarian function intact who were still producing their own testosterone reported significantly higher ratings of energy level and well-being than those women not receiving testosterone.

Having higher testosterone levels also gives us more energy to engage in physical exercise. Regular exercise is very beneficial since it increases our oxygen levels and promotes healthy circulation. This results in an increase in oxygen reaching the tissues and a greater production of beta-endorphins (natural mood elevators), both of which can potentially increase energy.

Because higher testosterone levels can increase strength, such an increase in physical ability can mean that a person finds exercise easier to do and is more likely to spend time in energy-generating physical activity.

Determination and Perseverance in Pursuing Goals

Testosterone levels in women, as in men, are associated with assertiveness and sexual drive. Women who report a higher libido are also more assertive in their behavior, often with a greater drive to achieve, and are usually busy, highly effective people.

However, during menopause, testosterone levels decline. About 30 to 50 percent of menopausal women experience a drop in libido soon after ceasing menstruation, because the ovaries stop making testosterone as well as estrogen. For others, the decline may be less rapid. This can have a significant effect on sex drive as well as the urge to achieve. I discuss this in more detail in the next chapter.

Many of my patients say that they suddenly feel as if something is missing in their relationship with their sexual partner, and that their interest in sex just evaporated after menopause. For these women, supplementing with testosterone can be of great benefit. Testosterone cream or the oral estrogen-testosterone combination therapy can significantly increase their sex drive. I share some research studies on this topic in the next section

A study cited in a review article appearing in the *Journal of Clinical Endocrinology and Metabolism* verifies this conclusion. Women who had had their ovaries surgically removed were injected with testosterone enanthate and reported an increase in the intensity of sexual arousal, sexual interest, and frequency of sexual fantasies above the effect they experienced taking only estrogen.

The Ability to Get Along With Other People

While estrogen therapy is often prescribed in postmenopausal women as a mood elevator, it is not the only hormone to produce this benefit. Research studies have shown that testosterone also has beneficial effects on emotional well-being, perhaps even more striking than those noted with estrogen replacement therapy (ERT). You might find this surprising but it has been verified by medical research.

For example, *The American Journal of Obstetrics and Gynecology* study cited above also examined the effect of testosterone on a variety of psychological symptoms. Patients completed a daily questionnaire, rating such items as feeling blue and depressed, crying spells, needless worry, and loss of interest in most things.

Those women receiving testosterone reported negative feelings significantly less frequently than women not receiving the hormone. If testosterone therapy is able to elevate mood in postmenopausal women, they are far more likely to get up in the morning with a seize-the-day attitude and participate fully in social and business activities.

6

Testosterone and Health in Women

Research studies show that testosterone relieves some of the symptoms of menopause and that it helps prevent osteoporosis. However, although this hormone seems to be protective of heart disease in men, high levels of testosterone may actually increase the risk of heart disease in women.

In clinical practice, testosterone is most often prescribed for women who complain that their libido seemed to evaporate with the onset of menopause. For these women, testosterone can restore their quality of life if they wish to remain sexually active.

Following are some health conditions that testosterone therapy may benefit in women who are in menopause.

Hot flashes, mood swings and insomnia

As you pass through menopause, you may experience a variety of symptoms initiated by the drop in hormone production that occurs at this time, including hot flashes, mood swings, and vaginal atrophy. Estrogen replacement therapy (ERT) is successfully used to treat many of these symptoms; there is also a growing body of clinical and experimental research that indicates that testosterone may be of benefit in reversing some of these symptoms, especially when combined with estrogen therapy.

A small study, reported in *American Family Physician* and presented at the sixth annual meeting of the North American Menopause Society, monitored two groups of women experiencing menopausal symptoms. One group of twelve women were each given 1.25 mg of estrogen daily, while a second group of thirteen women were each given the same dosage of estrogen and 2.5 mg of methyltestosterone. While both treatments had a positive effect on vaginal dryness and hot flashes, only the combined therapy helped relieve associated nervousness, irritability, fatigue, and insomnia. Other studies have shown that combined hormone therapy is also more effective in improving sleep quality and energy levels.

Loss of Libido

Testosterone levels in women are associated with sexual drive. As I indicated in the last chapter, your testosterone levels decline during menopause. About 30 to 50 percent of menopausal women experience a drop in libido soon after ceasing menstruation, because the ovaries stop making testosterone as well as estrogen. For others, the decline may be less rapid.

Many of my patients describe this decrease in desire as "something missing from their relationship with their sexual partner:' or that their interest in sex just evaporated after menopause. This speaks to the first of four phases of sexual response—desire. The other three—excitement, orgasm, and resolution—are equally important, and can be equally problematic if testosterone levels are low.

In these cases, many women say that pain during sex due to vaginal dryness and atrophy significantly decreases arousal. This is often due to decreased blood flow to the vaginal tissues, changes in lubrication, and shrinkage of the vagina itself, due to atrophic changes in the tissue. If you experience difficulties with either desire or arousal, orgasm may not readily occur.

Fortunately, supplementing with testosterone can significantly increase all three phases while estrogen treatment has not been found to be effective in reversing this decline

A study appearing in the *Journal of Clinical Endocrinology and Metabolism* cited several controlled studies documenting an increased intensity of sexual drive, sexual arousal, and frequency of sexual fantasies in women receiving testosterone supplementation. It also strengthens the tissues of the genital area, benefitting the vagina and vulva in women for whom fragility of these tissues has become an issue.

I have had a number of women patients who have been placed on testosterone therapy after a total hysterectomy (in which both the uterus and the ovaries are removed) or for the treatment of certain gynecologic conditions. Many of these women found that the testosterone therapy suddenly put their libido into high gear. These women reported that they thought and fantasized about sex constantly and requested frequent sexual activity with their partner if they were currently in a relationship.

Several of my patients told me that such intense sexual desire was a problem since their partners simply did not have the sexual stamina to keep up with their demands. This was particularly true for women in their fifties and sixties whose husbands' libidos were on the decline.

While replacement with estrogen and progesterone may be enough to control most menopause-related symptoms, it may not be effective in restoring libido. I have found that nothing matches testosterone for its effectiveness in restoring libido.

Testosterone is available through most pharmacies in either pill or cream form. Testosterone creams are sometimes used as a treatment for vaginal atrophy. It must be used carefully, however, because side effects of excessive androgen use can include masculin-ization such as deepening of the voice or growth of excessive facial hair.

Depression and Anxiety

While estrogen therapy is often prescribed in postmenopausal women as a mood elevator, it is not the only hormone to produce this benefit. Low levels of testosterone also impact your emotional well-being.

Studies have shown that testosterone has beneficial effects on emotional well-being, perhaps just as striking as those noted with estrogen replacement therapy. Additionally, testosterone may be even more effective than certain anti-depressants in lifting mood and managing depression in menopausal women.

This can have a life-changing impact. If testosterone is able to elevate mood, you are far more likely to get up in the morning with a seize-the-day attitude and participate fully in and enjoy family, social, and business activities.

Osteoporosis

The importance of androgens like testosterone in the development of the male skeleton is generally accepted, but scientists are now discovering that testosterone also plays a more important role in female bone health than was previously thought. The use of combined estrogen and testosterone therapy may be more effective at preventing osteoporosis than estrogen therapy alone. While estrogen slows down the rate of bone loss, testosterone helps promote formation of new bone. This can be of great benefit even for women in whom osteoporosis has already begun.

In one study, appearing in *Obstetrics and Gynecology*, sixty-six women who had undergone surgical menopause were given estrogen either alone or combined with testosterone. While both treatments prevented loss of bone in the spine and hip, only the combined therapy produced a significant increase in bone mineral density in the spine.

Arthritis

As you age, your testosterone production begins to decline. This can be bad news for your hips, knees, ankles, and wrists, as this hormone has a proven anti-inflammatory effect on the joints. In fact, according to a study from the *Annals of the New York Academy of Sciences*, people with rheumatoid arthritis have significantly decreased levels of testosterone (as well as pregnenolone and DHEA).

Even worse, as you enter mid-life, these declining hormone levels also thin the cartilage, tendons, and ligaments of your joints. As the muscles surrounding the joints try to help out your failing joints, they begin to clench and contract. This can lead to aches, pain, and stiffness throughout your entire body.

As the joints and surrounding muscles work overtime to compensate for this reduction in movement and ease, you begin to experience less flexibility and increased friction. This quickly sets the stage for increased wear and tear on your joints and the onset of arthritis. Testosterone therapy can be very beneficial in helping to combat arthritis.

Decreased Energy

Several studies have demonstrated that women taking just estrogen replacement have lower levels of energy than those who also use testosterone replacement. Additionally, women who engage in regular exercise have more energy because of it. This results in an increase in oxygen reaching the tissues and a greater production of beta-endorphins (natural mood elevators). Because higher testosterone levels can increase strength, such an increase in physical ability can mean that you find exercise easier to do and are more likely to spend time in energy-generating physical activity.

The Testosterone-Estrogen Health Problem

This is actually a pretty accurate description of polycystic ovarian syndrome (PCOS). If you suffer from PCOS, you can attest that it is a very frustrating and difficult condition. On one hand, you suffer with the effects of too much testosterone, including acne and increased growth of hair on the face, abdomen, upper thighs, chest, and back. Plus, you must contend with excess estrogen issues, such as infertility and menstrual irregularities. As if that wasn't bad enough, PCOS is also linked to insulin resistance, which can cause many sufferers to become severely overweight, and puts them at risk for developing diabetes.

Part of the difficulty of working with PCOS is that it has multiple underlying causes, namely a number of different hormonal imbalances. Specifically, the production of the pituitary's luteinizing hormone (LH) is significantly elevated in women with PCOS, while the production of the pituitary's follicle-stimulating hormone (FSH) is normal or slightly diminished. The imbalances in these hormones upset the normal production of estrogen, progesterone, and testosterone by the ovaries and adrenal glands, disrupting the healthy balance between all three of these sex hormones. Moreover, 50 percent of the women with PCOS have elevated levels of prolactin and decreased levels of dopamine.

In summary, women with many different types of menopause symptoms can benefit greatly from testosterone therapy, along with the other female hormones, estrogen and progesterone. These include hot flashes, insomnia, loss of libido, depression, anxiety, osteoporosis, arthritis and decreased energy.

I will be discussing many exciting and effective natural therapies to support your levels of testosterone and reduce the unpleasant symptoms of testosterone deficiency later on in this book.

7

The Cosmetic Effects of Testosterone Imbalance

In this chapter, I discuss two common conditions in which testosterone is a stealth culprit. If you suffer from either acne or facial hair it is likely that your levels of testosterone are probably out of balance and need to be brought under control.

Acne in Women

I've had many women come to me for advice in treating adult acne, even including several of my good friends! In addition to treatment options, many want to know why this teenage condition is plaguing them in their twenties, thirties, forties and even past midlife. The answer is simple. It is the same reason you broke out in your teens — hormones and stress.

The cause of acne can be found deep in your hair follicles. Each hair follicle has a sebaceous gland connected to it. This gland secretes sebum, an oil and wax mixture that keeps your skin moist and lubricated. During hormonal changes (such as puberty, menstruation, and perimenopause) and times of stress, you experience an increase in male hormones (androgen). This causes changes in the pH of the skin and overstimulates the sebaceous gland, which responds by secreting excess sebum. This in turn creates the skin lesions we call acne.

Acne can go through three stages. Blackheads are the first stage. They occur when sebum and oil block skin pores. Most of the oil in the pores is white, but the oil that is exposed to the air on the skin surface turns black. As the pore becomes clogged, bacteria mult-iplies and inflammation sets in, setting up stage two — whiteheads.

With this stage, the oil has no pore opening to the outside and drainage cannot occur. Cysts form underneath the skin and become infected. Your body responds to this by sending white blood cells to fight the infection. The result is a whitehead on the surface of the skin. If the cysts are too deep to be seen through the skin's layers, they can cause the third stage — cystic acne. These cysts are hard and deep and can be extremely painful to the touch.

In order to treat adult acne, I often recommend that women try a variety of approaches: diet, supple-ments, and topical treatments.

The first thing I recommend is to avoid refined sugar and foods high in sugar. Sugary foods over-stimulate the sebaceous glands and can trigger excess oil prod-uction. Refined sugar can also contribute to blood sugar imbalances, which can worsen symptoms of anxiety and stress, both of which can lead to break-outs.

Next, include vitamin A in your diet. It not only helps improve the overall health of your skin, it is especially helpful in suppressing oily skin and acne. In fact, one study found that high doses of vitamin A helped clear up even the most severe cases of acne in 90 percent of people treated with the vitamin. Since too much vitamin A can adversely affect liver function, I recommend that you take its water-soluble precursor—beta-carotene. Dosages between 15,000 and 25,000 III daily should provide you with adequate skin protection.

If you do break out, I suggest treating the blemish with tea tree oil. Its antiseptic properties have been used for centuries to clean and treat wounds. Even the early settlers of Australia and metal workers during the Second World War used this camphorous-smelling essential oil to treat cuts and insect bites. After washing the infected area, place one drop of Australian tea tree oil directly on blemishes. Read the product label carefully to be sure the oil contains 50 to 60 percent terpenes (preferably terpin-4-ol) and no more than 15 percent cineole. You can find tea tree oil in Whole Food Markets and most health food stores. A $5 jar will most likely last longer than your acne!

Finally, I suggest using blue light to treat breakouts. It is well known that sunlight is beneficial in clearing up acne. By isolating only the blue portion of the visible light spectrum and eliminating the potentially more dangerous invisible bands of ultraviolet light, blue light devices help clear up acne without negative side effects, such as sun burns, skin aging, cataracts, or increased risk of skin cancer.

The Growth of Facial Hair in Women

Another common occurrence related to testosterone imbalance, particularly too much, is the growth of facial hair. While changes in hair structure and growth are common during menopause, the unusual growth of darker, coarser hair in areas where hair may never have been before (chin, upper lip, chest, or abdomen) is due to the stimulation of hair follicles by low amounts of androgens. High estrogen levels block the action of these male hormones on hair follicle receptors.

However, after menopause, the effect of these low amounts of androgens is unmasked as your production of estrogen decreases. The development of facial hair occurs when the enzyme 5-alpha reductase (which exists in the facial hair follicles) converts all of this biologically active testosterone to a locally active form called dihydrotestosterone (DHT). DHT directly stimulates the follicle to switch from producing its usual baby-fine peach fuzz hair to the thick, dark facial hair that's associated with post-menopausal facial hirsutism.

Standard Treatment Options

Postmenopausal facial hirsutism is temporary and lasts until your body adjusts to its new hormonal composition—typically three to 10 years. Some women can get by with occasional tweezing during that adjustment period. But others find that they can't tolerate the facial hair, no matter how temporary it is.

Therefore, many women resort to all sorts of bleaches and depilatory creams to lighten or remove facial hair. However, these methods contain harsh chemicals that can irritate delicate facial skin. Another popular hair removal option is waxing, which temporarily (and painfully) removes all facial hair, including peach fuzz. While there's nothing particularly harmful about waxing, a lot of my patients have found that they simply do not like how different their face looks without that baby-fine peach fuzz. Plus, waxing can also be irritating to the skin.

Some women turn to electrolysis and laser treatments, thinking they are permanent solutions, but unfortunately, they are not. Using an electrical charge or a pulsed laser beam, these methods damage—but don't destroy—hair follicles. Electrolysis treats one follicle at a time, which is impractical for women who have a lot of facial hair. Laser treatment zaps a dime-sized area, but the beam targets dark pigment on the hair shaft, so it can't be used on light-colored hair or dark skin. Plus, it's painful and can cause burns and permanent skin discoloration. Not to mention, it typically takes 6 or more sessions to obtain noticeable results. According to David Larson, M.D., Professor and Chairman of Plastic and Reconstructive Surgery at the Medical College of Wisconsin, the hair usually grows back in about six months.

There is also a prescription cream available that helps reduce facial hair. It's called Vaniqa® (eflornithine hydrochloride), and it blocks the enzyme ornithine decarboxylase, which is involved in the synthesis of hair. However, the side effects — redness, stinging, burning, acne, or rash — make this option less than desirable.

More Options for Treating Facial Hair Growth

While all the treatments I have mentioned so far are viable options, they are not the best options because they can be painful, irritating, and in most cases, temporary solutions. However, the following strategies are free of side effects and address the underlying problem so that the growth of facial hair actually stops.

Because hair grows in cycles, these treatments require about two to three months of use before you see results. In the interim, you can remove the worst of the hair by plucking or sugaring. Like waxing, sugaring removes hair at the root, but it doesn't damage the surrounding skin. And it's painless!

I have often recommended to women the MOOM brand of sugaring. MOOM has only four ingredients: sugar, chamomile, lemon, and tea tree oil. While the sugar works to remove the hair, the tea tree oil acts as a mild anesthetic, and the chamomile and lemon function as natural antiseptics. Plus, MOOM is resin-free, hypoallergenic and a six-ounce jar lasts up to two months. For more information on MOOM, call 800-492-9464 or visit imoom.com.

There are also natural botanicals that, when used topically on the face, are known to inhibit 5-alpha reductase — the enzyme that activates testosterone in facial follicles. These substances have significant efficacy, especially when they're used together.

- Green tea extract (epigallocatechin gallate, or EGCG), a phytochemical from the green tea plant, inhibits 5-alpha reductase, and also has been shown to reduce skin inflammation in women suffering from rosacea.
- NDGA (nordihyroguaiaretic acid), an extract of chaparral, blocks receptor sites for 5-alpha reductase and also inhibits the skin's pro-inflammatory cascade.

- Zinc, azelaic acid, and vitamin B6: Even at low doses, zinc and azelaic acid (from the yeast Pityrosporum ovale) are potent 5-alpha reductase inhibitors because they work synergistically. Vitamin B6 enhances their activity and their ability to penetrate the skin. In one study, when very low doses of these agents were applied together, their combined activity blocked 5-alpha reductase by an amazing 90 percent.

Luckily, I have found a product called Acne Recover Repair Lotion Pod B that contains all five of these nutrients. It was developed by Dr. Randall Wilkinson, M.D. and sold through Trienelle Skincare (trienelle.com). If you'd like to order it, call the company at 800-539-5195 so they can adjust the packaging to exclude the rest of their acne treatment system.

8

Checking Your Levels of Testosterone

Before using testosterone therapy, it is important to have your levels tested to see if you have a deficiency. In this chapter, I share with you a very useful questionnaire that I developed that will help you to determine if you have symptoms or health conditions linked to testosterone deficiency for which testosterone therapy could be useful. I also discuss laboratory testing for testosterone.

Are You Testosterone Deficient?

The following checklists will give you an idea of whether you are experiencing the effects of inadequate testosterone production.

Quality of Life Indicators: If you answer yes to two or more indicators, you may have a testosterone deficiency; particularly if you are in menopause. Check any that pertain to you.

- o I suffer from persistent fatigue.
- o I lack stamina.
- o I have experienced a decline in my level of assertiveness.

- I typically have little desire to take risks.
- I have less interest than I used to in launching new projects and attempting new activities.
- I have a tendency toward depression.
- I often feel withdrawn.

Physical Indicators: If you answer yes to three or more of these questions, you very likely need to test your testosterone levels.

- I am over the age of fifty.
- I experience menopausal symptoms such as hot flashes, mood swings, and vaginal dryness.
- I lack interest in sex.
- I have a tendency toward depression.
- I often feel withdrawn.
- I have experienced a decline in the frequency of my sexual activity and orgasms.
- I suffer from persistent fatigue.
- I have osteoporosis and suffer from frequent bone fractures.
- I have rheumatoid arthritis.
- I lack stamina.
- I have experienced a decline in my level of assertiveness.
- I typically have little desire to take risks.
- I have poor muscle tone or weak muscles.

Testing for Testosterone Deficiency

Total testosterone production is somewhat difficult to assess, as the amount varies during the day, with higher levels occurring in the morning. Additionally, there are seasonal variations. Furthermore, a normal testosterone reading may mask a testosterone deficiency because the majority of testosterone in the bloodstream is bound to the protein SHBG and the protein carrier albumin.

Only about four percent of testosterone in the bloodstream is free, unbound and available to body tissues, where it can perform its functions. As you age, an increasing amount of testosterone remains bound, so in an older person, a normal reading of circulating testosterone does not necessarily indicate that adequate amounts of testosterone are available. Routine laboratory testing measures total hormone concentration, so special assays are required to measure the amount of active free testosterone.

When it comes to measuring testosterone, I highly recommend saliva testing, since the testosterone in the saliva is the type that is unbound. Best of all, saliva hormone testing is accessible. Even physicians who still don't routinely order saliva hormone testing will usually write an order when a patient requests it. You can even order a limited saliva hormone test kit on your own directly from a laboratory, without a doctor's order.

From 2 to 5 ml of saliva is needed. Samples remain viable for up to seven days but must be analyzed within that time. A person submitting a saliva sample must note the time of day it was taken, as hourly levels vary. Persons using testosterone creams applied to the skin may have very high readings. While testosterone blood levels can be tested through hospital and clinical laboratory facilities, saliva testing is currently also being done by specialized laboratories. Most of these laboratories require a physician's prescription in order to have testing done. There are also laboratories that will allow consumers to request their own sex hormone testing

If you think saliva hormone testing is right for you, consider consulting your physician. Having your doctor order the test has two advantages: The profile is more extensive, and your insurance may cover the cost. Several laboratories perform the test; in the event your physician does not have a preference, I recommend Genova Diagnostics (gdx.net or 800-522-4762), as well as ZRT Laboratory (zrtlab.com or 866-600-1636). If your doctor doesn't order the test, or you simply want insight to help you develop your own self-care regimen, you can order a test kit from several sources. Aeron Laboratories has a wonderful Life Cycles saliva test kit (aeron.com or 800-631-7900).

When testing testosterone levels, you will need to submit 2-5 ml of saliva. Samples remain viable for up to seven days, but must be analyzed within that time. A person submitting a saliva sample must note the time of day it was taken, as hourly levels vary. Also, if you are already using testosterone cream that you apply to the skin, you will likely have a very high reading.

Ranges of Testosterone Levels:

Blood: 20 to 80 ng/dL*
Saliva: 20 to 50 pg/mL**

If your results indicate that you are deficient in testosterone (or if you scored high on the checklists), there is a solution. Let's take a look at the many ways you can restore your testosterone levels safely and effectively, and start feeling better than ever!

*figures from MedlinePlus (a service of the US National Library of Medicine and the National Institutes of Health)

** figures from womenshealth.com

9

Restoring Testosterone

Over the years, I've had countless women of all ages come to me seeking ways to increase their sex drive, especially with the onset of menopause. As their levels of sex hormones diminish at midlife, including testosterone, women have told me that their interest in sex just seemed to "evaporate". As discussed in the previous chapters, low sex drive- along with low energy and vitality, and even osteoporosis-are linked to a deficiency in testosterone levels.

In this chapter, I share with you my program to help you restore your testosterone levels. I discuss how you can restore this critical hormone at the central nervous system level, with the help of key neurotransmitters, as well as powerful nutritional supplements and herbs. You'll also discover the role your ovaries and adrenals play in testosterone production, and how you can slow the breakdown of testosterone in the liver.

I also discuss nutrients that serve as hormone mimics that greatly help to restore such testosterone related functions like libido or sex drive. These include yang herbs and nutrients that help to promote nitric oxide production.

Restore Your Own Hormones

As with all hormones, testosterone production begins in the brain. In this section I talk about the amazing chemistry of the brain that promotes the production of testosterone within the body.

The Chemistry of the Brain

There are also three significant types of brain chemicals; neurotransmitters, neurohormones and neuropeptides which help to regulate our hormone production.

Neuropeptides are responsible for the cell-to-cell communication system in your body. A peptide is a short chain of amino acids connected together, and a neuropeptide is a peptide found in neural tissue. Neuropeptides are widespread in the central and peripheral nervous systems and different neuropeptides have different excitatory or inhibitory actions.

Neuropeptides control such a diverse array of functions in the body. When they work together properly, the wonderful results in your body include elevated mood and other positive behaviors and emotions, stronger bones, better resistance to disease, glowing skin, and boosted metabolism. Conversely, if your neuropeptides function abnormally, the result can be an increased tendency towards neurological and mental disorders such as Alzheimer's disease, epilepsy, and schizophrenia.

There are several types of neuropeptides. Some of the most common include endorphins and beta-endorphins. Endorphins are opiod peptides, meaning they have morphine-like effects within the body. They produce feelings of well-being and euphoria, and a rush of endorphins can lead to feelings of exhilaration brought on by pain, danger, or stress. Endorphins also may also play a role in memory, sexual activity, and body temperature.

Beta-endorphins are another form of opiod peptides, but they are stronger than endorphins. They are composed of 31 amino acids and work in the body by numbing pain, increasing relaxation, and promoting a general feeling of well-being.

While there are many, many hormones and hormonal interactions that occur in the brain and body, the most widely known neurohormone is melatonin. Melatonin is a hormone produced from serotonin and secreted by the pineal gland. Its secretion takes place at night and is inhibited by light. As such, it sets and regulates the timing of your body's natural circadian rhythms, such as waking and sleeping.

Unfortunately, as you get older, you produce less and less melatonin. This is due, in part, to menopause. Women who have poor sleep patterns, such as night shift workers, are also more likely to have decreased melatonin production.

Neurotransmitters are naturally occurring chemicals that relay electrical messages between nerve cells throughout your body. While all three types of neurochemicals are important for hormone and overall health, neurotransmitters are particularly important for the production of sex hormones.

In the aggregate, all three types of neurochemicals help to regulate the brain's endocrine glands, specifically the hypothalamus and pituitary gland. Your brain's hypothalamus regulates the production of all sex hormones. Specifically, the hypothalamus produces a precursor hormone called gonadotropin releasing hormone (GnRH). When it is released, it travels to your anterior pituitary gland, where it stimulates the secretion of the follicle stimulating (FSH) and luteinizing hormones (LH). These hormones then travel to your adrenals and ovaries, where they stimulate the production of androgens (male hormones), especially androstenedione and testosterone (as well as estrogen and progesterone).

Amino Acids that Help to regulate Neurotransmitter Levels and Testostrone

The neurotransmitters norepinephrine, epinephrine, dopamine, and serotonin regulate the hypothalamus' release of GnRH. Without proper production and balance of these neurotransmitters, you cannot have proper balance of the sex hormones, including testosterone.

This is critical, as the other major neurotransmitter pathway, inhibitory neurotransmitters (those in the serotonin pathway) help to calm us down as well as to eliminate insomnia and anxiety. The main inhibitory neurotransmitter precursor is 5-hydroxytryptophan (5-HTP) whose recommended dosage is 50-200 mg once or twice a day.

On the reverse side, the excitatory neurotransmitters; norephinephrine, dopamine, and epinephrine have powerful antidepressant effects. They also support arousal, alertness, optimism, zest for life, and sex drive.

The amino acids phenylalanine and tyrosine are precursors for these excitatory neurotransmitters. Phenylalanine is an essential amino acid that must be taken in through the diet, while tyrosine is produced from phenylalanine. Without proper levels of these nutrients, your norephinephrine, dopamine, and epinephrine levels will most likely be decreased. This can lead to low libido, depression, and other conditions also associated with low testosterone levels.

To ensure you have adequate levels of these vital amino acids, I recommend that you take either 500-1,000 mg of tyrosine per day or 500 mg phenylalanine once or twice a day. (Phenylalanine is a precursor of tyrosine.) In addition to taking it in supplement form, you can increase your levels of phenylalanine by consuming soybeans, fish, meat, poultry, almonds, pecans, pumpkin and sesame seeds, lima beans, chickpeas, and lentils.

Be sure to take tyrosine in divided doses, half in the morning and half in the afternoon. Do not take in the evening, as it may interfere with sleep. Also, I generally don't recommend going over 1,000 mg a day of tyrosine. Do not take tyrosine in conjunction with MAO inhibitors, and taper off if you start having headaches. Be sure to take phenylalanine and tyrosine with 25-100 mg of vitamin B6 and a small amount of protein.

Note: I strongly advise that you undertake a program to restore and properly balance your neurotransmitter levels under the care of a complementary physician, naturopath, or nutritionist. You should also have your neurotransmitter levels tested regularly, as dosage needs vary from woman to woman.

Herbs That Benefit Neurotransmitter Production and Testosterone

Mucuna Bean

Like phenylalanine and tyrosine, the tiny mucuna bean has also been shown to increase your libido and restore your sex drive. This power-packed legume can be traced as far back as medieval times, and was first described in the English literature in 1804. While every part of the plant is full of medicinal promise, the greatest benefits come from the seeds and root.

The key to mucuna's reputation lies in its rich store of L-dopa, one of the few natural sources of the precursor to dopamine, your brain's neurotransmitter responsible for energy, alertness, and libido.

As I indicated above, dopamine is normally made from the amino acids phenylalanine and tyrosine. Up until age 45, levels of dopamine remain fairly stable in your body. However, after 45, levels decrease by about 13 percent every 10 years.

The aphrodisiac qualities of mucuna have been known for centuries. In fact, it is one of two primary treatments for low libido in India. An animal study from the journal *Fitoterapia* confirmed this benefit. Researchers found that the mucuna bean can produce "striking improvement in normal mating behavior, potency, and libido and substantiates its use as a sexual function improver."

If you would like to try mucuna to put the pep back in your sex life, I recommend taking 300 mg/day in capsule form, standardized to 60 mg L-dopa. I am particularly fond of the Natural Path Center extract (naturalpathcenter.com or 608-826-9076), as well as the extract from NutriScience (nutriscienceusa.com or 203-334-3535).

Note: If you are currently taking antidepressant medications such as Zoloft or Prozac, you should check with your physician before using mucuna.

Another exciting area of research for mucuna involves Parkinson's disease, which is often characterized by symptoms such as muscular rigidity, resting tremor, slowness of voluntary movement, and difficulties with balance and walking. In the early 1920's, it was discovered that when dopamine levels were abnormally low, symptoms associated with Parkinson's began to appear.

As a chemical messenger between nerve cells, dopamine helps sensory and motor neurons communicate, thereby regulating motor coordination, muscle movement, etc. Without dopamine, these messages are not passed between the nerve cells, thereby resulting in Parkinson's disease.

Due to its high concentrations of L-dopa, researchers looked to the mucuna bean for a possible answer to this disease. In 1995, scientists gave a derivative of the mucuna bean (HP-200) to 60 Parkinson's patients for 12 weeks. Initial dosages were 7.5 grams of the herb derivative in powder form, mixed with water, and administered orally three times a day. The dosage was then increased at the second and fourth weeks. By the end of the study, the average daily dose was 45 grams of HP-200. At that time, researchers found that there was statistically significant improvement in the patients' conditions. The only adverse effects included nausea and vomiting in a few patients.

Tribulus Terrestris

Tribulus terrestris is a weedy, flowering plant native to warm temperate and tropical climates, such as those found in southern Europe and Asia, northern Australia, and Africa. Also known as cat's head, devil's thorn or devil's weed, puncture weed, Maltese cross, and Mexican or Texas sandbur, tribulus is most commonly used for its ability to boost testosterone levels by raising LH and GnRH levels.

As I have said in previous chapters, GnRH stimulates the production of LH, which stimulates the production of the androgenic hormones, including testosterone. By increasing GnRH and LH levels, tribulus allows you to enjoy the benefits of optimum testosterone levels (such as strong muscles and a healthy sex drive), without the risks associated with excess testosterone).

According to several studies, tribulus is highly effective in increasing both fertility and libido. One animal study found that tribulus increased sexual response in castrated rats. The rats experienced both increased mounting behavior, as well as greater blood flow to the penis. This benefit has also been seen in humans. Research has shown that women taking tribulus enjoyed both increased libido and enhanced emotional well-being.

To enhance testosterone production and increase libido, I suggest taking 100-200 mg of tribulus terrestris per day.

Maca

Maca, also known as Lepidium peruvianum or Lepidium meyenii, is one of the most traditionally used and valued Peruvian herbs. At one time, this malty, butterscotch flavored root was considered so valuable that the Incas limited its use to their royal court.

In the 1960's and 1980's, German and American researchers begin studying Peruvian botanicals, and were captivated with what they discovered. Due to its incredibly high nutrient content, maca soon became known as "the lost crop of the Andes."

Specifically, maca contains a number of minerals, vitamins, fatty acids, plant sterols, amino acids, and alkaloids, among other phytonutrients. Calcium makes up 10 percent of maca's mineral content. Magnesium, phosphorus, and potassium are also present in significant amounts. It contains smaller amounts of iron, silica, iodine, man-ganese, zinc, copper, and sodium. Maca also contains a number of vitamins and amino acids, including B1, B2, B12, vitamin C, vitamin E, and quercetin, as well as arginine, lysine, tryptophan, tyrosine, and phen-ylalanine.

Maca has been used for decades (if not centuries) to stimulate and regulate the endocrine system (adrenals, thyroid, ovaries, and testes); increase fertility; enhance libido; and increase energy, stamina, and endurance. However, it is most commonly known for its ability to increase sexual desire.

According to an issue of *Andrologia*, maca does improve sexual desire. In a double-blind, placebo-controlled study, researchers looked at different doses of maca as compared to placebo to determine if maca had an effect on sexual desire. They found that maca improved sexual desire within eight weeks of treatment, and that the desire was still present at 12 weeks.

Unlike Viagra, which works at a circulatory level, maca works at the hormonal level. That's why maca's use isn't limited to men. It has also been shown to improve sexual activity and satisfaction in women by increasing vaginal lubrication.

Maca can also be used to balance hormone levels. As an adaptogenic herb, maca can help to regulate hormones produced by glands in the endocrine system. Unlike conventional hormone replacement therapy (HRT) and even phytoestrogens, all of which work to mimic your body's hormones, maca helps your body produce its own unique balance of hormones. It does this by encouraging your ovaries and adrenals to produce the hormones you need, in the levels you need them, apparently more toward the progesterone and testosterone side of the equation.

This was shown in a study from the *Journal of Veterinary Medical Science*. Researchers tested the effects of maca on mouse sex hormones. They found that while progesterone and testosterone levels increased significantly in those mice that received the maca, their estradiol levels were not increased. In other words, the maca helped to raise the levels of progesterone and testosterone to offset the blood levels of estradiol.

If you are interesting in trying maca, a traditional dosage is 2-10 grams; however, dosages are unique to each woman, so you will need to determine which dosage works for you. There have been no acute toxic effects of maca, even at very high doses. In fact, many Peruvians eat it every day! I am fond of Whole World Botanicals' Royal Maca (wholeworldbotanicals.com or 888-757-6026).

Note: If you are naturally sensitive or allergic to herbs, you may want to avoid maca altogether, or at least use it cautiously. In any event, I suggest starting with the low end of the recommended dosage, as too much can cause increased hot flashes, breast tenderness, or headache. It is also recommended that you avoid maca if you have a hormone-related cancer (due to lack of formal studies), liver disease, if you are pregnant or nursing, or if you are currently taking conventional HRT.

Glandulars that Support the Brain and Testosterone Levels

Glandular therapy is also helpful in boosting testosterone levels. The success of glandular therapy lies in their ability to help restore hormone function by supporting the health of your endocrine glands themselves.

Glandulars are often comprised of purified extracts from the secretory endocrine glands of animals. Most commonly, extracts are drawn from the thyroid and adrenal glands, as well as the thymus, pituitary, pancreas, and ovaries. Most extracts come from cows, with the exception of pancreatic glandular preparations usually drawn from sheep.

In the past, experts believed that glandulars could not be effective because the intestinal lining of a healthy person was impenetrable, and that proteins and large peptides could not breach its barrier. However, recent evidence has shown that large macromolecules can and do pass completely intact from the intestinal tract into the bloodstream. In fact, there's further evidence to suggest that your body is able to determine which molecules it needs to absorb whole, and which can be broken down.

Both animal and human studies alike have proven this theory. In some cases, several whole proteins taken orally, including critical enzymes, have been shown to be absorbed intact into the bloodstream. Additionally, many smaller proteins and numerous hormones have also been found to be absorbed intact into the bloodstream, including thyroid, cortisone, and even insulin. In essence, it means that the active properties of the glandulars stay active and intact, and are not destroyed in the digestive process.

There are multi and single-glandular systems available from companies like Standard Process — a leader in the field. However, they do require a prescription from a health care practitioner. Other good products are also available in health food stores and should be used as part of a nutritional program to support healthy menstruation.

Examples of widely used and accepted glandulars involve the thyroid and the adrenals. Natural thyroid medications such as Armour Thyroid, Naturthyroid, and Bio-Thyroid have been the preference of complementary physicians for decades. Unlike many of the commonly prescribed brands of thyroid therapy that only replace a synthetic form of T4, these natural thyroid replacements contain the whole animal-derived thyroid gland, including T3 and T4. This is a significant difference. T3 is more physiologically active than T4, and is critical in regulating normal growth and energy metabolism. Without the use of glandulars, this type of natural thyroid replacement wouldn't be possible. However, the thyroid glandulars sold in the health food stores have the hormone removed and are used to support the function of your own gland.

Adrenal glandular preparations are even more common. With the stress epidemic in this country, the majority of Americans are walking around with depressed adrenal function. This can also manifest as fatigue, susceptibility to infection, allergies, and infection.

Fortunately, whole adrenal extracts have been found to help restore the health and function of comprised adrenal glands. They have also been shown to possess cortisone-like properties that help treat asthma, eczema, rheumatoid arthritis, and even psoriasis.

To help support healthy testosterone levels, I suggest taking a good multi-glandular or single glandular product from a company like Standard Process (standardprocess.com). These could include glandulars such as hypothalamus, pituitary, ovary, adrenal, and thyroid, depending on the specific needs of each individual woman.

I also highly recommend that you consider taking a whole brain glandular, if appropriate. To further support your adrenal function, I recommend taking 1,000-3,000 mg of a mineral-buffered vitamin C each day with a meal, 25-100 mg of a vitamin B complex a day, and an additional 250 mg of B5 (pantothenic acid) twice a day.

Testosterone Production in the Ovaries and Adrenals

In addition to stimulating testosterone production at the central nervous system level, you can also increase this vital hormone in your ovaries and adrenals with the help of certain important nutrients. I've found that DHEA, boron, and ginseng are critical for increasing testosterone production in your endocrine glands.

DHEA

DHEA is the precursor hormone to the major sex hormones testosterone and estrogen (but not progesterone). It is produced mainly by the adrenal glands, with smaller amounts also produced by the brain, skin, and ovaries. Once DHEA is produced by the adrenals, it travels through your bloodstream to cells throughout your body, where it's converted into testosterone, and then estrogen (in the form of estrone) in your adrenals and, subsequently, your ovaries and fatty tissues. Therefore, by increasing your DHEA levels, you can increase your body's production of testosterone.

If you choose to use DHEA, start with the lowest recommended dosage. It is better absorbed when taken with food and it's best to take it in the morning, because it can have a stimulating effect. Begin with a daily dosage of 5-15 mg in capsule form and monitor the effect. You can increase the dose by 5-10 mg each day, but do not exceed 25 mg daily.

Note: Before taking DHEA, have your hormone levels tested and consult an informed health care professional who can monitor your response to the hormone. Not all women are good candidates for DHEA therapy, as some may experience such side effects as anxiety and nervousness. Women should have a mammogram and Pap smear test done before starting DHEA supplementation to avoid the risk of stimulating a preexisting cancer of the reproductive tract, as DHEA will increase the levels of the major sex hormones.

JENNIFER'S STORY

When Jennifer came to see me, her most distressing complaint was her lack of libido and difficulty enjoying sex with her husband. She had gone through menopause at age 49, and now, one year later, she complained that her sex drive had not only evaporated, but intercourse was painful because her vaginal tissues would tear a bit during penetration. In addition to a powerful libido-enhancing nutritional program of DHEA, PABA, arginine, and other important nutrients, she began using bioidentical estrogen and progesterone, as well as testosterone creams to build up her tissues. Within no time, sex became much more pleasurable once again.

Boron

While the trace mineral boron is most commonly associated with increasing estrogen levels, it has been found to increase testosterone as well. This may be one reason it is so beneficial in the fight against osteoporosis.

According to a study published in *Nutrition Today*, boron reduced urinary excretion of calcium by 44 percent and significantly reduced excretion of magnesium as well. It also found that it increased levels of both testosterone and beta-estradiol.

To help boost testosterone levels and prevent osteoporosis, I suggest taking 3 mg of boron a day.

Ginseng

The herb ginseng has an almost legendary reputation for treating nearly every ailment known to man. In the 1950's, scientists began to test these claims and found that when high quantities of standardized extracts were administered, ginseng could be a very beneficial tonic and therapy. As an adaptogen, it has been shown to improve testosterone levels, and help maintain normal biological functions such as stamina and immunity.

The most widely used and studied type of ginseng is panax ginseng, which is either of Chinese, American, or Korean origin. When processed in its mature form, after at least six or eight years of growth, panax ginseng should contain 13 or more hormone-like compounds called ginsenosides. Clinical studies have shown that panax ginseng minimizes the harmful effects of stress on the body, protects against damage caused by radiation, and improves liver function.

Besides these actions, ginseng also has an effect on reproductive function. Traditionally, panax ginseng was taken to enhance virility and fertility. Human studies assessing this function have yielded mixed results, but animal studies, such as one published in the *American Journal of Chinese Medicine*, have demonstrated ginseng's ability to increase sexual and mating activity. Another study from the *Archives of Andrology* found that a five percent preparation of ginseng resulted in a significant increase in blood testosterone levels. Based on its traditional use and these modern studies, ginseng appears to be a suitable treatment to improve sexual function.

If you are interested in trying ginseng, I suggest taking 4-6 grams of a high-quality panax ginseng root per day. Ginseng and extracts of ginseng vary greatly in type and quality. The most valued are wild roots that are old and well formed, which have a high proportion of active substances. The lowest grade comes from the smaller roots of cultivated plants. They may contain various parts of the plant as well as additives. For this reason, it is important to use a standardized preparation that has guaranteed amounts of the active ingredients. The dosage is then based on the potency of the ginseng preparation being administered. As with many therapies, it is best to start with a small dosage and increase gradually. One regimen recommends taking ginseng on a repeating schedule, with two to three weeks of ginseng followed by two weeks with no treatment. Women do best on American or Chinese ginseng, as they are better suited for the female body.

Note: Side effects of ginseng include nervousness, hypertension, morning diarrhea, skin problems, insomnia, and euphoria. That's why it's important that you monitor yourself for these symptoms. Additionally, it's best to avoid red Korean ginseng, which is too heating and drying for most menopausal women.

Slow Down the Breakdown of Testosterone

In the same way you want to maintain your levels of circulating estrogen during menopause, you also want to preserve testosterone. One of the best ways to do this is by preventing the breakdown of the hormone in the liver. The fat-soluble B vitamin PABA (para-aminobenzoic acid) is a critical part of this plan. Studies indicate that PABA helps to safely and effectively slow down the breakdown of sex hormones, including testosterone, in the liver. Research has shown that higher levels of PABA are associated with better mood and outlook, better vaginal lubrication, and improved sex drive — all of which are also indicative of higher testosterone levels. In fact, PABA is the only vitamin that has been shown to increase libido! To restore libido and help impede the breakdown of testosterone, I recommend taking 400-500 mg of PABA a day.

10

Support the Effects of Testosterone with Hormone Mimics

In addition to increasing testosterone production and slowing down the breakdown of the hormone, you can also use nutrients that help boost libido and sexual responsiveness. Two highly effective ways to accomplish this is to use yang herbs or certain nutrients that promote the production of nitric oxide.

Herbs That Support Testosterone-Like Effects

Herbs have long been the province of traditional and folk medicine, but many Western doctors are just now paying attention to their many uses. In recent years, several major universities such as UCLA and Columbia have hosted conferences on how to incorporate both European and Chinese herbs into standard treatment protocols.

In my practice, I've used herbs to help improve a wide variety of hormone-related complaints. When it comes to using herbs to restore libido and sex drive (which are testosterone-supported health benefits), I've found that damiana, Rhodiola rosea, Siberian ginseng, and gingko biloba are the most effective. These herbs also contain a wide variety of chemicals that help you increase vitality and stamina, generate assertiveness, gain energy, boost libido and sexual responsiveness, ease anxiety, and even generate feelings of optimism.

Damiana

Damiana is a yellow, flowering bush indigenous to hot and humid climates such as Central America, Mexico, and the southwestern U.S. It has a long history as an aphrodisiac for women, dating all the way back to the Mayan civilization. Women typically use the leaves to make a libido-lifting elixir to drink before intercourse.

In recent times, damiana has been used to increase sex drive and treat impotence. While no clinical trials have been performed on this herb, animal studies have shown that it does increase sexual desire and frequency of sex. Additionally, most herbalists agree that the alkaloids found in damiana are responsible for this mild, testosterone-like effect on the body.

The recommended dosage is 100-200 mg of damiana per day. To date, there are no known negative interactions or side effects associated with the herb.

Rhodiola Rosea

Rhodiola rosea is a popular plant indigenous to Eastern Europe and Asia. The ancient Greeks used the herb medicinally as far back as 100 A.D. Named for the rose-like odor of the rootstock when newly cut, Rhodiola rosea has been used for centuries in China to prolong life and enhance wisdom. Siberian healers believe that people who drink Rhodiola tea on a regular basis will live to be more than 100 years old. And in the former Soviet Union, Rhodiola has been used to diminish fatigue and increase your body's resistance to stress.

Rhodiola works to support testosterone (and other hormone production) by easing stress and fatigue, both killers of healthy hormone production. According to the journal *Phytomedicine*, Rhodiola is effective in fighting stress-induced fatigue. In one study, researchers tested 40 male medical students during exam time to determine if the herb positively affected physical fitness, as well as mental well-being and capacity. The students were divided into two groups and given either 50 mg of Rhodiola rosea extract or a placebo twice a day for 20 days.

Researchers found that those students who took the extract had a significant decrease in mental fatigue and increase of psychomotor function, with a 50 percent improvement in neuromotor function. Plus, scores from exams taken immediately after the study showed that the extract group had an average grade of 3.47, as compared to 3.20 for the placebo group.

To ease fatigue, stress, or anxiety, all of which can play havoc with your testosterone production, and boost your energy and stamina (which testosterone supports), I recommend 50-100 mg of Rhodiola rosea three times a day, standardized to 3 percent rosavins and 0.8 percent salidrosides.

While the herb is generally considered safe, some reports have indicated that it may counteract the effects of antiarrhythmic medications. Therefore, if you are currently taking this type of medication, I suggest you discuss the use of Rhodiola rosea with your physician.

Ginkgo Biloba

The ginkgo biloba tree originated about 250 million years ago, and a single tree can live as long as 1,000 years. It is often planted in urban settings, lining fashionable streets and decorating parks, as it resists disease, insects, and pollution.

Modern science is finding that this ancient plant has a wide range of benefits, including improving blood flow, preventing the brain from aging, and improving all four stages of sexual response—desire, excitement (lubrication), orgasm, and resolution. It has even been shown to reverse sexual dysfunction in women taking certain antidepressants.

When it comes to helping improve blood flow, there is no debate as to ginkgo's benefits. Three hundred published scientific papers and 40 double-blind studies have proven its efficacy. This is due, in large part, to the rich store of antioxidant bioflavonoids found in ginkgo. This also allows this amazing herb to help improve circulation and fight inflammation in just about every organ system in the body, as well as scavenge free radicals.

As for your brain health, ginkgo increases blood flow and energy production, as well as improves production of neurotransmitters, chemicals that help transmit nerve signals. Plus, ginkgo protects brain and nerve cells from deteriorating by stabilizing cell walls and scavenging free radicals that can destroy delicate cell structures. It also helps maintain the brain's supply of energy in the form of glucose and oxygen. This is beneficial, as it supports healthy neurotransmitter and brain-based hormone production.

I suggest taking 30 mg of Ginkgo biloba extract (standardized to 24 percent flavonoid glycosides and 6 percent terpene lactones) three times a day. Ginkgo is extremely safe and side effects are uncommon.

Spice Up Your Sex Life

Studies have shown that certain scents have particularly strong aphrodisiac-like qualities, especially cinnamon, cloves, ginger, and nutmeg. In addition to using these spices when cooking, place potpourri or essential oils that include these scents in your bedroom, bathroom, or wherever tickles your fancy.

Keep in mind that these herbs support the yang in Chinese medicine. They are heating and drying. Therefore, if you are having hot flashes, vaginal dryness, etc., you should not use these herbs. Conversely, if you are bloated, carry excess weight, and need to "contract:' then these spices are just what the doctor ordered.

Cinnamon—When the Crusaders returned to Western Europe from the Far East, they brought a reputed sexual stimulant with them—cinnamon. Today, this spice is one of the most common herbs across the globe.

Cloves—The Persians, Egyptians, Europeans, and Arabians all considered this spicy scent to be an aromatic aphrodisiac. In the Sudan, women concoct a wedding potion that consists of clove mixed with musk, cherry, and sandalwood. They then wear the blend to the party so its aroma will drift in the air as they dance the night away.

Ginger—The ancient Persian physician Avicenna used to mix this fragrant spice with honey as a cure for impotence. Whether its benefits are due to its pungent aroma or its ability to increase circulation, ginger soon grew to be known as the spice of "burning desire' Today, women in Senegal wear ginger in their belts in order to attract men, while female New Guineans can't say no to a man who emits ginger's strong scent.

Nutmeg—While this spice has a strong smell, it is actually a relaxing scent that relieves anxiety and stress, and even reduces blood pressure. The Chinese are particularly fond of nutmeg's aphrodisiac qualities. They have found that it can elicit a feeling of rapture and invigoration. In North America in the 1700's, men and women often added nutmeg to their nightcaps. Maybe our ancestors were onto something!

Promote Nitric Oxide Production

Another way to further support the effects of testosterone in your body and promote healthy sexual functioning is to promote the production of nitric oxide. Nitric oxide is a gaseous molecule produced in the body from the amino acid arginine. As a potent vasodilator, nitric oxide enhances the flow of blood through the arteries and veins to all the tissues and cells of your body. It not only improves the health and functional capability of your heart, but also helps to support the health of your respiratory, neuroendocrine, immune, reproductive, and other systems because of its beneficial effect on circulation.

Impaired circulation due to diminished nitric oxide production can also lead to diminished physical and mental energy and immune-system function, diminished sexual responsiveness, poor or slow recovery from exertion and injury, and impaired wound healing. Furthermore, levels of nitric oxide tend to decrease with age. In fact, high nitric oxide producers typically have healthy skin and hair and well-developed muscles. In contrast, elderly individuals (and even younger individuals with diminished nitric oxide production) often have thinner hair and paler, thinner skin. Nitric oxide is particularly important for healthy sexual function and responsiveness.

In my experience, there are five key nutrients that promote nitric oxide production: arginine, citrulline, ginseng, alpha lipoic acid, and vitamin C.

Arginine

L-arginine, an amino acid found primarily in protein sources such as red meat, dairy products, eggs, poultry and fish, is used within your body to produce nitric oxide. As a result, it helps to promote blood flow and vascular relaxation, and works to make tissues firmer and more elastic. In fact, research studies have shown that intravenous administration of arginine can increase nitric oxide production.

Additionally, a nutraceutical research and development company has been able to orally administer small amounts of arginine combined with other nutrients, allowing the body to increase its production of nitric oxide.

The L-arginine/nitric oxide pathway has been shown to be responsible for sexual arousal and heart protection. While most of the research surrounding L-arginine and sex drive has been focused on men, there have been a few intriguing studies involving women.

In one randomized, double-blind, placebo-controlled, three-way crossover clinical trial, 23 women with documented Female Sexual Arousal Disorder (FSAD) were given L-arginine (as well as a few other nutrients) for six months. The women were shown a non-sexual movie, as well as a sexual film. The degree of each woman's sexual reaction was documented by changes in vaginal pulse amplitude. The women also filled out a self-report questionnaire. Researchers found that women taking the L-arginine had a significant and rapid increase in vaginal pulse amplitude response after watching the sexually charged film.

In a separate study presented at the *Ninth Annual Congress on Women's Health & Gender-Based Medicine*, researchers determined that L-arginine increased sexual desire and satisfaction. This double-blind, placebo-controlled study looked at 93 women between the ages of 22 and 73, all of whom reported a lack of sexual desire. Half of the group was given L-arginine daily, while the other half received a placebo. After four weeks, 64 percent of the women taking L-arginine reported improved satisfaction with their sex life, and 64 percent reported greater sexual desire.

I can also speak to the positive effects L-arginine has on sex drive that I've seen in my own practice. In one case, a 38-year old woman began taking this amino acid to help regulate her periods. On a subsequent appointment, she told me that her libido was stronger since she started taking the supplement. Another patient taking L-arginine described an increased intensity during sex, a sensation she attributed to the nutrient.

Not only does it improve the health and functional capability of the heart and boost libido, but arginine also helps to support the health of the respiratory, neuroendocrine, immune, reproductive, and other systems because of its beneficial effect on circulation.

If you would like to try L-arginine, I recommend taking 1,000 mg in capsule form once or twice a day, in combination with 250 mg of B5 and 250 to 350 mg of choline once a day to promote better blood flow to your organs and tissue. L-arginine is readily available in most health food stores.

Note: Women taking lysine for a serious herpes infection should avoid supplemental use of L-arginine, as it may counteract any potential benefits of the lysine. Additionally, women with diabetes may want to check with their physicians before using L-arginine, as it may interfere with insulin and carbohydrate metabolism.

Citrulline

Another amino acid — citrulline — also increases nitric oxide production, thus relaxing blood vessels and improving blood flow. Latin for watermelon (from which the nutrient was first discovered), citrulline is needed by your liver to detoxify ammonia.

In fact, citrulline is produced from a combination of ammonia and carbon dioxide. The byproduct (ornithine) is then combined with aspartic acid, and later metabolized into arginine.

Beyond its nitric oxide-producing effects, citrulline also increases energy and boosts your immune system. To receive all of these benefits, I suggest taking 500-1,000 mg of citrulline a day.

Other Key Nutrients

While they play a much lesser role, the antioxidants alpha lipoic acid and vitamin C help to fight free radical damage that may occur with increased nitric oxide production.

Alpha lipoic acid (ALA) is a universal antioxidant, working in both water and fat-soluble parts of your cells. It recycles other antioxidants in your body and scavenges more types of free radicals than any other known antioxidant.

Similarly, vitamin C is an important antioxidant. It not only helps prevent the oxidation of "bad" low-density lipoprotein (LDL) cholesterol and increases "good" high-density lipoprotein (HDL), it also helps maintain vitamin E levels and helps absorb iron. Plus, vitamin C has an antihistamine effect, meaning that it may shorten the length and severity of infections, including colds. Vitamin C is also plays an important role in the production of glutathione, a powerful substance that helps to increase nitric oxide production.

Most importantly, ALA and vitamin C work synergistically to protect you from free radical damage. One study in particular from the *International Journal of Cosmetic Science* looked at the effects ALA and other antioxidants had on women with sun damage. They gave the women either a supplement that contained 5 mg of ALA, 10 mg of vitamin E, 90 mg of vitamin C, and 6 mg of lutein, or a placebo. After two months, the women who took the antioxidant-rich supplement had lower levels of free radicals in their blood, as well as better skin hydration than women who took the placebo.

To receive the full benefits of these outstanding antioxidants, I recommend taking 50-100 mg of ALA and 500-3,000 mg of a mineral-buffered vitamin C per day, in divided doses.

11

Supplementing With Testosterone

The final step in my program is to supplement your nutrient regimen with natural, biochemically identical testosterone, if needed, for the "heavy lifting" that the use of actual hormone replacement therapy provides. Now that estrogen and progesterone hormone replacement therapy has become more generally accepted, countless numbers of women have also begun to supplement with testosterone.

At about age 20, a woman produces peak levels of estrogen, progesterone, and testosterone, but by the time she reaches midlife and passes through menopause, production of these hormones is greatly diminished. To remedy this, estrogen and progesterone are routinely prescribed to restore a woman to youthful hormone status. However, testosterone, which was very much a part of her original hormonal makeup, is much less commonly added into the mix.

Among those women who do decide to take this hormone, the most common reasons are its ability to help prevent vaginal discomfort and soreness while increasing sex drive. In my practice, I've seen testosterone rapidly restore libido (though not for all women), which is an issue for many of my patients, as it affects the pleasurable aspects of intimate relationships. Testosterone is also prescribed for postmenopausal women who are troubled by abnormally low body weight, poor musculature, poor coordination, and osteoporosis.

Physicians who practice conventional medicine pre-scribe testosterone in the form of capsules. However, there are other forms of testosterone to consider, including testosterone creams and gels.

Synthetic Testosterone

The two forms of synthetic-testosterone admin-istration for women are by capsule and subdermally.

Capsules

The synthetic androgen methyltestosterone has been used clinically for many years. Taken orally as a capsule, the product name is Android®, from ICN Pharmaceuticals. Each capsule contains 10 mg of the hormone. Replacement therapy starts at 10 mg a day and can be gradually increased, with a limit of 50 mg per day.

Testosterone is also marketed combined with estrogen, in a product called Estratest®. The full-strength capsule contains 1.25 mg of esterified estrogen and 2.5 mg of methyltestosterone. There is also a half-strength capsule. Combined estrogen-testosterone therapy is not appropriate for all women. It is probably most useful in women who have undergone surgical removal of their ovaries or whose ovaries have stopped producing even small amounts of testosterone and estrogen soon after menopause. Estratest is recommended for more short-term use, to treat moderate to severe hot flashes associated with menopause. The hormone replacement should be taken for three weeks on and one week off. Medication should be stopped or reduced at three- to six-month intervals.

The drawback of orally administered testosterone is that it is poorly absorbed once in the digestive tract. Another option is subdermal testosterone.

Subdermal Administration

While this delivery method is more common for men, some women have had testosterone pellets implanted beneath the skin. These contain 75 mg of testosterone USP and provide sustained release of the hormone. One pellet can be used for three to six months.

Natural, Bioidentical Testosterone

Natural testosterone is produced by compounding pharmacies, which are able to formulate a wide range of dosages. These can be prepared as a cream or a gel (the two most popular forms), or as sublingual tablets or oral capsules.

Creams

Most women's health-prescription compounding pharmacies suggest using creams containing 0.5 mg/g to 1 mg/g of testosterone. One-quarter teaspoon provides 1 g of cream and 0.5 mg of testosterone. A typical dose is 1/8-1/4 teaspoon, used daily in the morning. The cream is applied to various sites, which are rotated, including the inner thigh, the back of the hand, the abdomen, and the arm. An advantage of testosterone cream is that, once absorbed through the skin, it immediately enters the general circulation and travels directly to target cells. Only later does the testosterone pass through the liver, which then begins to metabolize, or break down, the hormone.

Gels

The gel is normally applied to vaginal tissue, from which the testosterone is absorbed into the bloodstream.

Sublingual Tablets

Sublingual tablets are well absorbed. Women usually begin with doses of 2-5 mg, but even a dose of only 0.5 mg may be sufficient. A reduced dose may be appropriate for a woman who is also taking estrogen, because estrogen activates testosterone receptor sites and strengthens its hormonal effect.

Oral Capsules

Capsules can be prepared with no preservatives, which some people prefer. However, capsules do have a disadvantage in that, once absorbed, the testosterone must first pass through the liver before entering the general circulation. Because the liver metabolizes the hormone, a smaller quantity of less active testosterone reaches target cells.

Injections

In a double-blind, placebo-controlled trial of 107 women with active rheumatoid arthritis, weekly supplemental testosterone injections brought significant improvement in comfort and quality of life (November 1996, *Annals of the Rheumatic Diseases*).

Positive research on Bioidentical Testosterone

As you can imagine, much research has been done on the use of supplemental testosterone. Unfortunately, most of this research is performed using synthetic versions of the hormone. However, I and other like-minded alternative and complementary medicine physicians believe that biochemically identical testosterone has the same benefits found with the synthetic versions, but is a healthier hormonal option.

One study published in the *American Journal of Obstetrics and Gynecology* found that women who had received a total hysterectomy, including removal of their ovaries, benefited greatly from testosterone supplementation. As the ovaries make one-third of the testosterone in the female body, their removal causes a significant decline in testosterone production. The women were divided into four groups and given combined estrogen and androgen, one or the other of the hormones alone, or a placebo. The treatments were administered for three months, followed by a differing treatment for another three months. There was also a control group of ten women who underwent hysterectomy, but retained their ovaries. The women receiving androgen therapy, alone or with estrogen, and the women with ovarian function intact reported significantly higher ratings of energy and well-being than those women not receiving androgens.

Another study cited in a review article appearing in the *Journal of Clinical Endocrinology and Metabolism* found that testosterone cream or the oral estrogen-testosterone combination therapy can significantly increase sex drive. Women who had had their ovaries surgically removed were injected with testosterone enanthate (a synthetic) and reported an increase in the intensity of sexual arousal, sexual interest, and frequency of sexual fantasies above the effect they experienced taking only estrogen.

Similarly, a study from the *Journal of Clinical Endocrinology and Metabolism* cited several controlled studies also documenting an increased intensity of sexual drive, sexual arousal, and frequency of sexual fantasies in women receiving testosterone supplementation.

Additionally, testosterone has a positive effect on a variety of psychological symptoms. In a study from the *American Journal of Obstetrics and Gynecology*, patients completed a daily questionnaire, rating such items as feeling blue and depressed, crying spells, needless worry, and loss of interest in most things. Those women receiving testosterone reported negative feelings significantly less frequently than women not receiving the hormone.

Research from the journal *Menopause* confirms these findings. The study tested the effects of a SSRI (selective serotonin reuptake inhibitor) antidepressant versus a combination of various hormonal therapies. Researchers divided 72 postmenopausal, depressed women into four groups. One group received the antidepressant alone, another received the antidepressant with a synthetic estrogen-progesterone combination, the third took a synthetic testosterone with the antidepressant, and the fourth received a combination of all four drugs.

At the end of 24 weeks, only 48 women were still involved in the trial. Of the remaining women, researchers found that they all enjoyed relief from their menopausal symptoms. However, only those women who took the antidepressant with the testosterone reported an improvement in mood.

Testosterone supplementation can also improve your physical health, including menopausal symptoms and osteoporosis. A small study reported in *American Family Physician* and presented at the sixth annual meeting of the North American Menopause Society, monitored two groups of women experiencing menopausal symptoms. One group of 12 women were each given 1.25 mg of estrogen daily, while a second group of 13 women were each given the same dosage of estrogen and 2.5 mg of methyltestosterone. While both treatments had a positive effect on vaginal dryness and hot flashes, only the combined therapy helped relieve associated nervousness, irritability, fatigue, and insomnia. Other studies have shown that combined hormone therapy is also more effective in improving sleep quality and energy levels.

In another study from *Obstetrics and Gynecology*, 66 women who had undergone surgical menopause were given estrogen either alone or combined with testosterone. While both treatments prevented loss of bone in the spine and hip, only the combined therapy produced a significant increase in bone mineral density in the spine.

Be Cautious on Dosage

The downside of supplementing with testosterone is that, when taken in high amounts, masculinization can occur. Your voice may deepen, you may develop more facial hair, and there may be clitoral enlargement. Acne may develop, and existing skin problems can worsen. You may also experience changes in your menstrual cycle, and if you are pregnant and take testosterone, a female fetus can develop male sexual characteristics. However, these effects are not likely to happen when testosterone is administered in the smaller, safer dosages appropriate for women.

There is also a possibility that testosterone may increase your risk of heart disease, and if taken with estrogen, testosterone may neutralize some of the benefits of estrogen therapy. Testosterone lowers "good" HDL cholesterol, a risk factor for cardiac problems. There is some evidence that testosterone given by injection, rather than given orally, is able to maintain more healthful levels of HDL.

It is important for anyone taking testosterone to be monitored closely by a physician so that any adverse effects can be recognized and dealt with promptly.

Summary of Testosterone Therapies

Maintaining optimum testosterone levels not only improves your libido and enhances your mood; it also protects your heart and bones. By following the program I've outlined in the last two chapters, you can maintain proper testosterone balance for years to come.

1. Support testosterone production at the central nervous system level with tyrosine, phenylalanine, macuna, Tribulus terrestris, maca, and glandulars.
2. Support testosterone production in the ovaries and adrenals with DHEA, boron, and ginseng.
3. Slow the breakdown of testosterone in the liver with PABA.
4. Use herbs such as Damiana, Siberian ginseng, Rhodiola rosea, and Ginkgo biloba to support the effects of testosterone in your body.
5. Boost nitric oxide production with arginine, citrulline, alpha lipoic acid, and vitamin C.
6. Using biochemically identical natural testosterone.

About Susan Richards, M.D.

Dr. Susan Richards is one of the foremost authorities in the fields of family medicine and alternative medicine. Dr. Richards has successfully treated many thousands of patients emphasizing alternative health and integrative medicine in her clinical practice. Her mission is to provide her patients with safe and effective alternative therapies to greatly enhance their health and well-being.

A graduate of Northwestern University Feinberg School of Medicine, she has served on the clinical faculty of Stanford University School of Medicine and taught in their Division of Family and Community Medicine.

Her Facebook page, Dr. Susan's Healthy Living, has over one million followers. She is also an ordained minister and her ministry receives over a million prayer requests for healing each year.

NOTES

NOTES

NOTES